Simple an

Copycat Recipes

The cookbook of famous restaurants in your home.
Learn to cook like celebrity chefs using the best recipes from Cracker Barrel, Red Lobster and more.

Jaqueline Weber

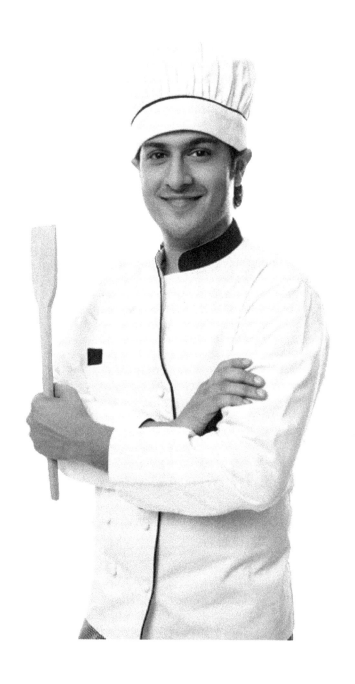

TABLE OF CONTENTS

—

INTRODUCTION

One of the most common questions I get is if it's okay to copycat recipes from other people. This is a difficult question to answer because there are several factors that will determine whether or not you can use someone else's recipe.

Copycat recipes have many advantages over original recipes. They are cheaper, they're easier to make, and they taste better. Also, copycat recipes are not copyrighted and therefore you can share them with others for free.

Copycat recipes are a great way to save money and time when cooking at home. The key is to make sure that you are getting the most bang for your buck when it comes to ingredients.

Copycat recipes are a great way for you to get creative with your food and be more adventurous in the kitchen. Making your own recipes can help you save money, and they don't have to be complicated. Copycat recipes are a great way to learn how to cook with ingredients you may not be familiar with. You can get creative and make something unique, or you can follow a recipe and make the dish exactly as it's written. Copycat recipes are a great way to save money and their benefits are numerous.

Copycat recipes are a great way to save money and still get the results you're looking for. This recipe is copied from Reddit, and it's been a hit ever since.

Copycat recipes are great for people that want to try something new but don't have the time or energy to make something from scratch. The recipes in this book are simple and can be made in less than 30 minutes. Copycat Recipes benefits your business by giving you the opportunity to make money. When you're starting out, or even if you're an established company, you can use copycat recipes to get your name out there and drive traffic to your website.

Darlene's copycat recipes are an essential part of the 5 Second Cheesecake brand. Not only do they help her make a quick and easy dessert, but they also give her brand instant credibility. One of the biggest advantages of copycat recipes is that they save you time. Almost all of us are busy and some, especially moms and students, have very limited time in a day. Copycat recipes are a great way to save time and money in the kitchen. You can whip up healthy meals for your family in no time with our copycat recipe's roundup. All you need is a little inspiration.

Copycat recipes are the best way to get new consumers interested in your brand. If you have a hit product, it can be easy to keep everyone happy by producing and selling a copycat version. Copycat recipes are a great way to simplify your cooking and save money. If you're a food blogger or cook, it's important to share your recipes with others in order to gain more followers and exposure. Copycat recipes are great for the following reasons (bolded ones are my favorites): Inexpensive and you can make a lot of them. They're easy to make, especially if you already have the ingredients on hand. 3.

Copycat recipes are not plagiarism, instead they are a way to learn how to make delicious meals. These recipes are especially helpful for those who do not have a cookbook and want to make something tasty and healthy. Copycat recipes are a good way to save money and show customers how much you love their favorite foods. Copycat recipes are a great way to save money and make at home beauty products. This saves you time and money by not having to buy products that you can easily make at home. There are also tons of recipes that look absolutely delicious.

ITALIAN RECIPES

Primavera Skillet

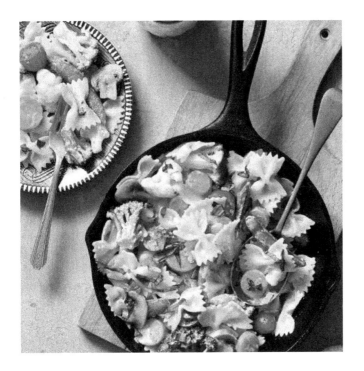

Preparation Time: 15 minutes

Cooking Time: 30 minutes

Servings: 4 (2 pizzas)

Ingredients:

- 1 lb. of pizza dough (or refer to recipe for Pizza Pretzel for homemade pizza dough recipe)
- 1/2 head of broccoli, florets separated
- 1/4 red onion, sliced thinly
- 2 bell peppers, sliced lengthwise
- 1 cup of cherry tomatoes
- 1 cup of ricotta
- 1 cult of shredded mozzarella
- Salt & pepper to taste
- A pinch of rosemary
- A pinch of thyme
- 1/4 cup of crumbled Feta cheese
- Olive oil for drizzling
- Flour to coat a working space

Directions:

1. Preheat the oven to 400ºF.
2. Prepare a baking sheet by drizzling the surface with olive oil. Lay the peppers, onion, broccoli, and tomatoes onto the tray and season with salt and pepper. Toss the contents on the tray and give it a good shake, to mix the vegetables with the oil and seasoning. Sprinkle some rosemary and thyme over some of the vegetables. Place the tray in the oven and let it roast for 18-20 minutes.

3. While the vegetables are roasting, prepare the pizza base. Get another oven-proof skillet/baking tray and drizzle more olive oil on the surface.

4. Lightly flour a working space and roll the dough out onto the workspace. Divide the dough into two equal parts, then using a rolling pin, roll each ball of dough into a circular shape, about 12" in diameter.

5. Place one of the pizza bases onto the baking tray/skillet and brush both of the pizza bases with olive oil.

6. Dollop a spoonful of ricotta in the center of both of the pizza bases and spread it evenly, leaving about 1" around the circumference (as this is now the crust). Then, generously sprinkle mozzarella over the bases.

7. Once the vegetables have roasted, remove them from the oven and raise the oven temperature to 500ºF.

8. Evenly spread the vegetables onto the pizzas, then season once more with salt. Finally, crumble Feta cheese over the tops.

9. You can use the second tray (which the vegetables were roasting on) to place the second

pizza on, and bake both pizzas simultaneously, or you can bake them individually.

10.   Pop the pizzas in the oven for about 12 minutes, until the cheese has melted and the crust is golden.

Nutrition: Calories 333 Carbohydrates26.8g Fat 16.6g Protein21.5g

Antipasto Salad

Preparation Time: 10 minutes

Cooking Time: 5 minutes

Servings: 6

Ingredients:

For the salad:

- 2 large romaine hearts, chopped thinly
- 1/2 cup of sliced olives
- 1/2 lb. salami, sliced thinly
- 8 oz. of mozzarella balls, cut in halves
- 1 cup of quartered artichoke hearts
- 1/4 cup of mint leaves
- 1 cup of cherry tomatoes, chopped in halves
- 1 cup of chopped pepperoncini (banana peppers are a good substitute)

For the homemade vinaigrette:

- 1/2 cup of olive oil
- 1 tsp mustard seeds
- 1/4 cup of red wine vinegar
- 1 tsp of Dijon mustard
- 1/2 tsp of oregano
- 1/2 tsp of chili flakes
- Salt & pepper to taste

Directions:

1. Mix the lettuce, salami, artichokes, mozzarella, tomatoes, pepperoncini, olives, mint, and artichoke in a large salad bowl. If you have salad spoons, use this to mix the contents together; if not, toss the contents in the bowl to have them integrate with each other.

2. For the vinaigrette, take a jar or container (anything that has a lid) and combine all of the ingredients: olive oil, mustard seeds, red wine vinegar, Dijon mustard, oregano, and chili flakes, and season with salt and pepper to taste. Stir the contents gently with a spoon/stirrer and close the container.

3. When serving the salad, stir the vinaigrette prior to drizzling over the salad (as the contents may have separated).

Nutrition: Calories 379 Carbohydrates3.9g Fat 34.6g Protein 14.5g

MAIN RECIPES

Bonefish Grill Copycat Bang-Bang Shrimp

Preparation Time: 10 minutes

Cooking Time: 35 minutes

Serving: 10

Ingredients:

- 1 1/4 cups of mayonnaise, low fat
- 5/8 cup of chili sauce, Thai sweet
- 7 1/2 dashes of garlic-chili sauce
- 2 1/2 lbs. of shrimp, peeled
- 1/2 cup of corn starch
- 4 leaves of lettuce
- 1/4 cup of green onion, chopped

Directions:

1. Pour in sweet chili sauce and mayo together in large sized bowl. Add garlic-chili sauce. Stir well. Spread the corn starch into wide, shallow dish. Press the shrimp into corn starch, giving it a fairly thin layer of coating. Heat oil in deep-fryer to 350F.

2. Deep-fry the shrimp in small batches till not transparent in middle anymore, five minutes or so per batch. Drain on plate lined with paper towels. Combine shrimp and mayo sauce in sauce bowl. Stir, coating shrimp well.

3. Line medium bowl using leaves of lettuce. Add shrimp to bowl. Garnish with the green onions. Serve.

Nutrition: 400 Calories 28g Total Fat 23g Protein

Black Angus Steakhouse's BBQ Baby Back Ribs

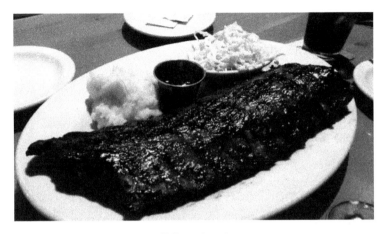

Preparation Time: 30 minutes

Cooking Time: 6 to 8 hours

Servings: 1

Ingredients

- 1 rack of pork ribs
- Your favorite barbecue sauces
- Onion powder, to taste
- Garlic powder, to taste

Marinade:

- 2 tablespoons kosher salt
- 2 tablespoons paprika
- 4 tablespoons granulated garlic
- 1 tablespoon onion powder
- 1 teaspoon cumin seeds

- 1 teaspoon Durfee Ancho pepper
- 2 teaspoons dry mustard
- 2 teaspoons black pepper

Rib Mop:

- 1 cup red wine vinegar
- 1 tablespoon garlic
- 1 cup water
- 3 tablespoons soy sauce

Directions:

1. Mix all of the marinade ingredients together. Rub the marinade all over the ribs to soak them in flavor.

2. Barbecue the meat over indirect heat at 250F to 300F for 3 to 4 hours. Add soaked fruit wood to the coals for additional aroma. Make sure that the temperature remains at 250F to 300F for the entire cooking duration. While the meat is cooking, mix together the rib mop ingredients in a bowl.

3. After three to four hours, transfer the meat to an aluminum pan and brush both sides with the rib mop.

4. Cook the ribs for another hour and then remove them from heat and mop them again. Continue cooking the ribs for another 3 to 4 hours, basting

them with the mop and some barbecue sauce every hour. When the ribs are done barbecuing, sprinkle them with onion and garlic powder before wrapping them in aluminum foil. Let the ribs rest for 30 minutes.

5. Situate the ribs to a plate and serve.

Nutrition: 1500 Calories 30g Total Fat 14g Protein

Texas Road House's Mesquite Grilled Pork Chops with Cinnamon Apples

Preparation Time: 40 minutes

Cooking Time: 40 minutes

Serving: 2

Ingredients

Cinnamon Apples:

- 4 apples (peeled, sliced)
- 2 tablespoons butter, melted
- 1/3 cup brown sugar
- 2 tablespoons lemon juice
- ¾ teaspoon cinnamon

Pork Chop:

- 2 pork loin chops with bone, room temperature; 2 inches thick

Paste:

- 2 tablespoons extra virgin olive oil
- 2 tablespoons Worcestershire sauce
- 2 teaspoons black pepper, cracked
- 2 teaspoons chili powder
- 2 teaspoons granulated garlic powder
- 2 teaspoons kosher salt
- 1 teaspoon cumin, ground

- ½ teaspoon cinnamon, ground
- Mesquite wood chips, drenched in water for at least 30 minutes

Directions:

1. Prepare the apples by cooking all the cinnamon apple ingredients in butter until the apples soften. When they are ready, set the cooked apples aside. Reheat before serving.
2. Before you begin with the meat, you need to:
3. Soak the mesquite chips as instructed; Leave the pork loin at room temperature for 30 to 45 minutes; and Preheat the grill on high.
4. Thoroughly mix all the paste ingredients together. When the paste is done, spread it over the pork chops, covering them completely. Take out chips from the water and place them in an aluminum foil pan.
5. Place the pan directly over the fire from the grill and cook the pork loin on both sides for about 6 minutes. Once seared, set the heat to medium. Place the pork over indirect medium heat and cook for another 25 minutes. Remove the pork from heat, wrap it in aluminum foil, and let rest for another 5 minutes. Transfer the pork to a

plate with the reheated apples. Serve the entire dish.

Nutrition: 316 Calories 22.5g Total Fat 20.5g Protein

Panda Express's Grilled Teriyaki Chicken

Preparation Time: 5 minutes

Cooking Time: 20 minutes

Servings: 4

Ingredients

- 2 pounds chicken thighs
- 2 tablespoons canola oil
- 2/3 cup sugar
- ¼ cup low-sodium soy sauce
- 1 teaspoon lemon juice
- ½ teaspoon garlic powder
- ¼ teaspoon ground ginger
- 1/3 cup water
- 2 tablespoons cornstarch dissolved with 2 tablespoons water
- Sliced green onions for garnish

Directions

1. Incorporate chicken thighs and canola oil and let sit until the grill is hot. Situate the chicken in a grill pan and grill for about 5 minutes on each side.

2. In a mixing bowl, combine the sugar, soy sauce, lemon juice, garlic powder, ground ginger and water. Heat to boiling, then decrease heat and simmer for 3 minutes. Stir in the cornstarch slurry and cook on low heat until the sauce thickens.

3. Spoon sauce over grilled chicken to serve. Sprinkle with sliced green onions.

Nutrition: 452 calories 10g Carbohydrates 23g Protein

Panda Express's Sweet Fire Chicken Breast

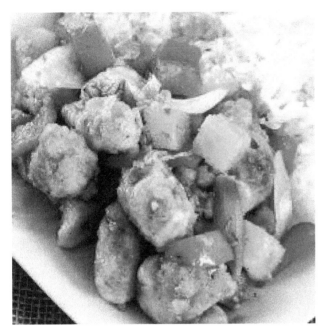

Preparation Time: 15 minutes

Cooking Time: 15 minutes

Servings: 4

Ingredients

- 3 large chicken breasts, cut into 1-inch pieces
- 1 (10-ounce) bottle sweet chili sauce
- 1 medium onion, sliced
- 1 large red bell pepper, chopped
- 1¼ cup pineapple chunks
- ¼ cup pineapple juice

- 2 cloves garlic, minced
- 1 cup all-purpose flour
- 2 eggs, beaten
- Oil for frying
- 2 tablespoons oil, if needed
- Salt and pepper to taste

Directions

1. Incorporate flour, salt and pepper to a shallow dish. Dip the chicken pieces in the beaten egg followed by a dip in the flour to coat. Set aside.
2. Cook oil in a large skillet over medium-high heat. When hot, add the chicken pieces and cook until golden brown on all sides, about 6 minutes.
3. Once done, pull out chicken from the skillet and place on a paper-towel-lined plate to drain excess oil.
4. If needed, mix in rest of the oil to the skillet and heat over medium-high heat. When hot, stir in onions, garlic and peppers and cook until the onions and peppers start to soften.
5. When soft, return the chicken to the skillet along with the chili sauce, pineapple and pineapple juice and allow to cook for about 7 minutes, stirring occasionally. Serve with a side of rice.

Nutrition: 624 calories 11g fats 31g protein

Panda Express's Black Pepper Chicken

Preparation Time; 20 minutes

Cooking Time: 15 minutes

Serving: 4–6

Ingredients

- 6 boneless, skinless chicken thighs
- 1 green bell pepper, diced
- 1 yellow onion, sliced
- 3 celery stalks, sliced
- 2 tablespoons cornstarch
- 1 tablespoon garlic powder
- ½ tablespoon black pepper
- ½ tablespoon onion powder
- 1 teaspoon ginger powder
- 2 tablespoons peanut oil
- 2 cups cooked rice

Sauce

- ½ cup chicken broth
- ¼ cup oyster sauce
- ¼ cup rice wine vinegar
- ½ tablespoon garlic, minced
- 1 teaspoon black pepper

- 1 teaspoon chili powder
- ½ teaspoon ginger powder

Directions

1. Combine all of the sauce ingredients, stir, and set aside. Dice the chicken into 1-inch pieces. Stir in cornstarch, salt and pepper to a mixing bowl. Toss the chicken in the mixture to coat.

2. Cook oil over medium-high heat in a large skillet. Cook the chicken in batches to keep the pieces from touching. This lets the individual pieces cook faster and brown more easily.

3. Once all of the chicken is browned, put it back to the skillet along with the vegetables and cook for about 5 more minutes. Add the sauce to the chicken and vegetables and allow to simmer for 10–12 minutes. Serve with rice.

Nutrition: 704 calories 10g fats 30g protein

Panda Express's Zucchini Mushroom Chicken

Preparation Time: 15 minutes

Cooking Time: 10 minutes

Servings: 4

Ingredients

- 1-pound boneless skinless chicken breasts, cut into bite-sized pieces
- 3 tablespoons cornstarch
- 1 tablespoon canola oil
- 1 tablespoon sesame oil
- ½ pound mushrooms, sliced
- 1 medium zucchini
- 1 cup broccoli florets
- ¼ cup soy sauce
- 1 tablespoon rice wine vinegar
- 2 teaspoons sugar
- 3 cloves garlic, minced
- 2 teaspoons minced ginger or ½ teaspoon ground ginger
- Sesame seeds, for garnish (optional)

Directions

1. Add the cornstarch to a shallow dish and season with salt and pepper. Add the chicken and toss to coat. In a large skillet, heat both the canola and sesame oil over medium high-heat. When hot, add the chicken and cook until brown on all sides.

2. Pull out chicken from the skillet and turn the heat to high. Cook the zucchini, mushrooms, and broccoli until they begin to soften, about 1 minute. Cook the garlic and ginger a bit longer. Continue to cook until the mushrooms and zucchini have softened to taste, then stir the chicken back into the skillet. When the chicken has heated up, stir in the soy sauce and the rice wine vinegar. Serve with rice.

Nutrition: 701 calories 11g fats 29g protein

Panda Express's Orange Chicken

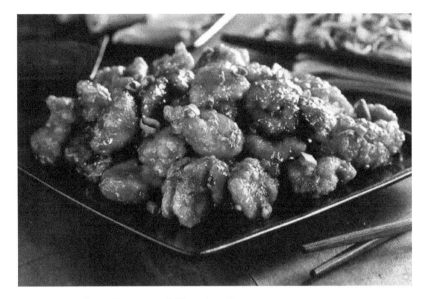

Preparation Time: 15 minutes

Cooking Time: 10 minutes

Servings: 4–6

Ingredients

- 1 egg
- 1½ teaspoons salt
- White pepper to taste
- Oil for frying
- 2 pounds boneless skinless chicken
- ½ cup cornstarch
- ¼ cup flour

Orange sauce

- 3 tablespoons soy sauce

- ¾ cup orange juice
- ½ cup brown sugar
- Zest of 1 orange
- 1 tablespoon oil
- 2 tablespoons ginger, minced
- 2 teaspoons garlic, minced
- 1 teaspoon red chili flakes
- ½ cup green onion, chopped
- 2 tablespoons rice wine
- ½ cup water
- 2 tablespoons cornstarch
- 1 teaspoon sesame oil

Directions

1. In a shallow dish, combine the ½ cup of cornstarch and the flour. In a second shallow dish, beat together the egg, salt, pepper and 1 tablespoon of oil. In a large skillet or deep saucepan, heat oil to 375°F.

2. Soak chicken pieces in the egg mixture followed by the flour mixture. Shake off any excess flour. Situate coated chicken to the hot oil and cook for about 4 minutes or until nicely browned. Transfer the chicken from the hot oil to a paper-towel-lined plate to drain.

3. Scourge soy sauce, orange juice, brown sugar and orange zest. In another skillet or wok, heat 1 tablespoon of oil. When hot, add the ginger, garlic, red pepper flakes and green onions. Cook for 1 minute.

4. Stir in the rice wine and soy sauce mixture. Cook for about 1 more minute, then add the chicken. Make a slurry with the water and remaining cornstarch and gradually add to the skillet until the sauce thickens. Add sesame oil to taste. Serve with rice.

Nutrition: 725 calories 12g fats 34g protein

PF Chang's Orange Peel Chicken

Preparation Time: 10 minutes

Cooking Time: 30 minutes

Serving: 4

Ingredients

- 4 boneless, skinless chicken breasts
- ¾ cup flour
- ¼ cup orange peel from 1 orange
- 2 tablespoons cornstarch
- 2 tablespoons garlic, minced
- 2 teaspoons black pepper
- 2 teaspoons Creole seasoning
- 2 teaspoons garlic powder
- 2 teaspoons onion powder
- 1 teaspoon chili powder
- Extra-virgin olive oil
- Orange peel sauce
- 1 cup tomato sauce
- 6 tablespoons orange juice
- 6 tablespoons chicken broth
- ¼ cup brown sugar
- 2 tablespoons sriracha
- 1 tablespoon soy sauce
- 1 teaspoon chili paste
- ¼ teaspoon black pepper

Directions

1. Peel and clean an orange, removing the white pulpy part and cutting out the segments which will be used for garnish. Julienne the peel and set aside with the segments. Incorporate all of the sauce ingredients in a mixing bowl. Set aside.

2. Cut the chicken into bite-sized cubes. Mix all of the spices. Toss over the chicken pieces. Stir to make sure the chicken is properly covered.

3. Mix flour and cornstarch. Pour over the seasoned chicken and stir again to make sure the chicken is coated.

4. Cook olive oil in a large skillet over medium-high heat. When hot, stir in the chicken and cook until browned on all sides. Once all cooked, take it from the skillet.

5. Pour in bit more olive oil to the pan, then toss in the orange peel slices and the garlic and cook just until garlic is fragrant. Add the sauce to the skillet and bring to a boil, then reduce heat and cook for 5 minutes. Situate chicken back to the skillet and cook for 5 more minutes. Garnish with orange segments and serve with rice

Nutrition: 691 calories 10g fats 31g protein

P.F. Chang's Crispy Chicken

Preparation Time; 20 minutes

Cooking Time: 2 hours

Serving: 4

Ingredients

Chicken

- 1-pound chicken breast, boneless, skinless, cut into medium sized chunks
- Vegetable oil, for frying and deep frying

Batter

- 4 ounces all-purpose flour
- 2½ ounces cornstarch
- 1 egg
- 6 ounces water
- 1/8 teaspoon baking powder
- 1/8 teaspoon baking soda

Chicken seasoning

- 1 tablespoon light soy sauce
- 1/8 teaspoon white pepper
- ¼ teaspoon kosher salt
- 1 tablespoon cornstarch

Sauce

- ½ cup sake or rice wine
- ½ cup honey

- 3 ounces rice vinegar
- 3 tablespoons light soy sauce
- 6 tablespoons sugar
- ¼ cup cornstarch
- ¼ cup water

Directions:

1. Mix the batter at least 2 hours in advance. Mix all the batter ingredients together and refrigerate. After an hour and 40 minutes, mix all the seasoning ingredients together and mix in the chicken. Make sure that the chicken is covered entirely.

2. Place the chicken in the refrigerator to marinate for at least 20 minutes. Incorporate all the sauce ingredients together - except the cornstarch and water - and set aside.

3. Before you begin frying your chicken:

4. Place a paper towel on a plate in preparation for draining the oil; and Heat your oil to 350F.

5. When your oil is heated, remove the chicken from the refrigerator and pour the batter all over it.

6. One by one, lower the coated chicken pieces into the heated oil. Keep them suspended until the batter is cooked, about 20 to 30 seconds.

7. When all the chicken is cooked, place it on the plate covered with the paper towel to cool and drain. Bring the sauce mixture to a boil. Though waiting for it to boil, incorporate the cornstarch and water in a separate bowl.

8. Slowly pour the cornstarch mixture into the sauce and continue cooking for 2 minutes, until the sauce thickens. When the sauce thickens, remove it from heat.

9. When the chicken is cooked, pour some sauce over the entire mixture, just enough to cover the chicken. Transfer everything to a plate with rice or Chinese noodles and serve.

Nutrition: 679 calories 12g fats 32g protein

SNACK RECIPES

Reese's Peanut Butter Cups

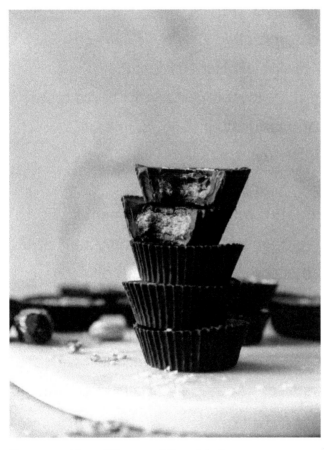

Preparation Time: 49 minutes

Cooking Time: 41 minutes

Servings: 4

Ingredients:

- Chocolate layers
- cup of dark chocolate (sugar-free)
- 1/2 tbsp. of vanilla extract (optional this should also be divided)
- 5 tbsp. of coconut oil
- Layers of peanut butter:
- 2 tbsp. of coconut oil
- 1/8 tsp. of vanilla extract (optional)
- 2 tsp. of artificial sweetener erythritol (to taste)
- 1 1/2 tsp. of peanut flour
- Salt to your taste

Direction

1. Cover muffin tin with parchment paper cut to their size. Temper the chocolate, only half of it. Heat the half of the coconut oil over boiling water, over the stove for the lower part chocolate sheet, constantly stirring, until melted. Tempering can also be done in the microwave, but with 20 seconds pauses, Add only half the vanilla quantity, if necessary

2. Fill the cups made of parchment paper bottom equally with chocolate 2 tsp. of worth, in every single one. Let it for freeze for ten minutes before the surface is solid, at least

3. Meanwhile, warm coconut oil, peanut butter in a bowl over boiling water or in a microwave for the peanut butter coating (same process as stage 2). Add the peanut flour, powdered sweetener, vanilla flavor, and salt if using, until smooth. If needed, add sweetener and sea salt to your liking

4. A tbsp. of the mixture of peanut butter is spooned over the chocolate coating to each cup's middle. It will expand into a circle a bit, but it does not yet touch the sides, which is what you want. Freeze for another 10 minutes, before the surface is solid, at least

5. In the meantime, make the top layer in chocolate. Heat in a bowl over boiling water or in a microwave, the procedure is the same as before the remaining chocolate and coconut oil that will be two and a half tbsp. remaining. Add the remainder of the vanilla (1/4 tsp.), if necessary.

6. Pour the chocolate in the ramekins over each peanut butter (almost 2 tsp.). The chocolate on the peanut butter sides' circle should fill the open room, and even cover the rim

7. Put back into the freezer for almost half an hour, before completely solid. Store it in the fridge

Nutrition 340 Calories 12g Proteins 14g Fat

Keto Pumpkin Pie from Maui Pie

Preparation Time: 32 minutes

Cooking Time: 3 hours

Servings: 16

Ingredients:

Crust:

- 3 tbsp. of coconut flour
- 1 1/2 cup of almond flour
- 1/4 tsp. of baking powder
- 4 tbsp. of butter melted
- 1 beaten egg
- 1/4 tsp. of Kosher sea salt

Filling:

- 1/2 cup of keto-friendly packed sugar
- 3 large eggs, beaten
- 1 cup of heavy cream
- 1 tsp. of ground cinnamon
- 1/2 tsp. of ground ginger
- 1/4 tsp. of ground nutmeg
- 1 cap of pumpkin puree
- 1/4 tsp. of ground cloves
- 1/4 tsp. of kosher sea salt
- 1 tsp. of pure vanilla extract
- Whipped cream

Direction

1. Let the oven preheat to 350F
2. Whisk the almond flour, sea salt, coconut flour, and baking powder in a big pot. Add the melted butter and egg, and then mix until dough develops. Place dough in a 9 "pie plate uniformly, and use a fork to poke holes all over the top
3. Bake for 10 minutes, until slightly yellow
4. Whisk pumpkin, cream, brown sugar, eggs, spices, and vanilla together in a large bowl until soft. Place the mixture of pumpkin into pre-baked crust
5. Bake for 45 to 50 minutes until filling is mildly jiggly in the center and crust is golden
6. Switch the oven off, and open the door panel. Let the pie cool for 1 hour in the oven, then refrigerate until ready for serving
7. If needed, serve with whipped cream

Nutrition 232 Calories 25g Proteins 10g Fat

Keto Tortilla Chips

Preparation Time: 24 minutes

Cooking Time: 32 minutes

Servings: 4

Ingredients:

- 2 cups of shredded mozzarella
- 1 cup of almond flour
- 1 tsp. of kosher sea salt
- 1 tsp. of garlic powder
- 1/2 tsp. of chili powder
- Freshly ground black pepper

Direction

1. Let the oven preheat to 350F
2. Use parchment paper to cover two big baking trays
3. Melt mozzarella in a microwave-safe bowl for around one minute and 30 seconds. Add the almond flour, garlic powder, sea salt, and chili powder and freshly ground black pepper. Knead the dough a couple of times with your fingertips before smooth ball forms
4. Place the dough between two sheets of parchment paper and fold out into a 1/8" thick

rectangle. Slice the dough into squares, using a knife or pizza cutter

5. Place chips on lined baking sheets and bake for 12 to 14 minutes, until the sides are golden and start to crisp

Nutrition 150 Calories 25g Proteins 8g Fat

Keto Copycat Ice Cream from Coconut Glen's

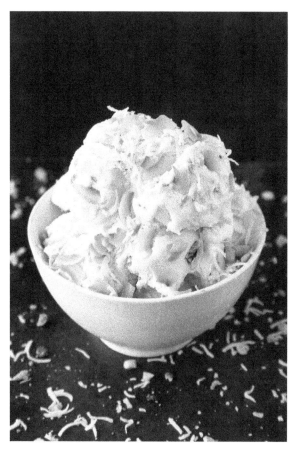

Preparation Time: 61 minutes

Cooking Time: 0 minutes

Servings: 3

Ingredients:

- 1 tsp. of pure vanilla extract
- 2 cups of whipping cream

- 1/4 cup of keto-friendly sugar (your choice)
- 2 caps of coconut milk
- A pinch of salt

Direction

1. For at least three hours, chill the coconut milk chill in the refrigerator, preferably overnight
2. To make whipped coconut in a big bowl, add coconut cream, leaving the liquid in the pan, and make whipped cream of coconut mix it with hand-mixer. Put it aside
3. To make whipping cream, beat heavy cream until soft peaks develop, but do it with a hand mixer, in a separate large bowl would be easy. Beat in Vanilla and Sweetener
4. Now mix whipped coconut with whipped cream by lightly folding, then move the mixture to a loaf saucepan
5. Freeze for around 5 hours, or until it becomes solid

Nutrition 262 Calories 5g Proteins 8g Fat

Snickerdoodle Truffles

Preparation Time: 19 minutes

Cooking Time: 29 minutes

Servings: 24

Ingredients:

Truffles:

- 1/2 cup of sugar (keto-friendly)
- 6 tbsp. of melted butter
- 1 tsp. ground cinnamon
- 1/4 tsp. of salt
- 1 tsp. of vanilla extract
- 2 cups of almond flour
- 1 tsp. of cream of tartar

Coating

- 1 tsp. of ground cinnamon
- 3 tbsp. of granular keto-friendly sugar

Direction

1. Whisk together the almond flour, Swerve, tartar cream, cinnamon, and sea salt in a large bowl. Incorporate melted butter and vanilla extract before the dough comes together. If the dough is too crumbly to hold together, apply a spoonful of water, and fold in

2. Scoop the circular tbsp. dough out and press a couple of times into your palm to help keep it together and shape it into a ball. Put on a baking sheet lined with waxed paper and repeat with remaining dough

Coating:

1. Whisk both the granular sugar and the cinnamon together in a small dish. Roll out the truffles until completely coated with the layer
2. Its 24 truffles, around. Two Truffles for each portion

Nutrition 250 Calories 18g Proteins 10g Fat

Ikea Swedish Meatballs

Preparation Time: 12 minutes

Cooking Time: 21 minutes

Servings: 2

Ingredients:

- 1 beaten egg
- 4 tbsp. of grass-fed butter
- 2 1/2 cups of minced beef
- 1/2 tsp. of Kosher sea salt
- 1/4 tsp. of black pepper
- 1/4 tsp. of all spices
- 1 piece of onion
- 1 1/2 tsp. of arrowroot powder
- 1/4 tsp. of nutmeg
- 1/4 tsp. of garlic powder
- 1/2 cup of heavy cream
- Olive oil
- 1-2 cups of beef broth
- 1/4 cup of almond flour
- 1/4 of crushed pork rinds
- 1 tsp. of Dijon mustard
- Mashed cauliflower
- Berry jam

Direction

1. In a pot or oven, melt a spoonful of butter over medium heat. Stir in the onion, a pinch of sea salt and sauté until it starts caramelizing (6-8 minutes). Take off heat and set aside to cool

2. Add to a wide bowl the minced Beef, almond flour, oil, seasoning, sea salt, spices, cooked onion and egg, and 2 tbsp. of heavy crème. Using your palms, combine all thoroughly and shape into circles

3. Heat up a bit of olive oil over medium heat in your pan, then cook the meatballs until all-over brown and cooked. You are going to want to move them around several times so that they cook uniformly. Move to a pan, then cover with foil when preparing the sauce

4. Add the rest of the butter to the skillet and cook until brown. To deglaze the pan, pour in the broth, remaining heavy cream, and mustard. Let it cook for a few minutes, then create a slurry with your preferred thickener (blend it with a couple of tsps. with cold water before adding it to minimize clumping). Continue to cook until the sauce already starts thickening and feel the seasoning

5. Put the meatballs back into the pan, cook for a few more minutes and serve immediately on cauliflower rice or any other rice of your choice

Nutrition 330 Calories 21g Proteins 10g Fat

Cheesecake Factory's Hamburger Patties with Creamy Tomato Sauce and Fried Cabbage

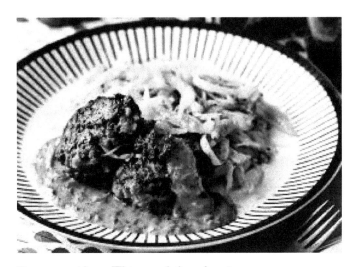

Preparation Time: 14 minutes

Cooking Time: 32 minutes

Servings: 4

Ingredients:

For Hamburger:

- 1/2 beaten egg
- 6 cups of minced beef
- 1/8 cup of parsley
- 1/2 tsp. of sea salt
- 1/8 tsp. of ground black pepper
- 1/2 tbsp. of olive oil
- 1 tbsp. of butter

- 1/2 cup of crumbled feta cheese

Direction

1. Add all of the hamburger ingredients to a big bowl. Blend it with a wooden knife. Do not over-mix because it will cause the cakes to become hard. Using moist hands to shape eight long patties
2. Add olive oil and butter to a large frying pan
3. Fry for at least 10 minutes over medium-high heat, or until the patties have developed a nice color. Flip them after a few minutes so both sides can be equally cooked
4. Whisk the tomato paste and the cream together in a small bowl
5. Put the mixture to the skillet when the patties are cooked completely. Allow it to simmer and stir occasionally
6. Season with sea salt and black pepper
7. Right before serving sprinkle parsley
8. Green cabbage (fried in butter)

For Gravy preparation

- 2/5 cup of whipping cream
- 3 tbsp. of fresh parsley
- 1 tbsp. of tomato paste
- Sea salt

- Black pepper
- Fried Green Cabbage
- 1 1/2 cup of shredded green cabbage
- 2 tbsp. of butter
- Sea salt
- Black pepper

Direction

1. Thinly cut the cabbage using a sharp knife
2. Add butter to a big frying pan
3. Put the pan over medium-low heat and sauté the thinly sliced cabbage for a minimum of 15 minutes, or until wilted and lightly browned from edges
4. Stir constantly and reduce the heat a little at the end. Garnish with sea salt and black pepper

Nutrition 200 Calories 22g Proteins 10g Fat

Wendy's Beef Chili

Preparation Time: 21 minutes

Cooking Time: 49 minutes

Servings: 4

Ingredients:

- 1/2 cup of diced tomatoes
- 3 tbsp. of chili powder
- 1 tsp. of black pepper
- 2 diced onion
- 1/4 of Kidney Beans drained
- 2 tsp. of cumin
- 1 cup of beans
- 8 cups of minced beef
- 1 tsp. of sugar
- 1/4 cup of diced celery
- 1/4 cup of diced bell black pepper
- 1 tsp. of sea salt
- 1/2 tsp. of oregano
- 2 tsp. of garlic powder
- 2 cups of water

Direction

1. Sauté minced beef and drain it
2. To remove more fat, add water, simmer and drain
3. Place in a big pot and add all the ingredients

4. Let it boil, lower the heat, stir every 15 minutes, cover, and simmer for 2-3 hours

Nutrition 300 Calories 14g Proteins 7g Fat

Fudpuckers Bacon-wrapped Tuna

Preparation Time: 19 minutes

Cooking Time: 34 minutes

Servings: 4

Ingredients:

- 4 finely sliced of bacon
- 2 cups of Tuna fillets
- 1/4 cup of Worcestershire sauce
- 1/2 cup of soy sauce
- Black pepper
- Sea salt to taste
- 4 tbsp. of honey

Direction

1. To secure the bacon into Tuna, an easy way to wrap Tuna is to use a toothpick to secure Tuna's bacon
2. Put the grill on. To make a basting sauce, mixing honey, soy sauce, and Worcestershire sauce.
3. Rub this mix on Tuna
4. Start cooking the bacon-wrapped Tuna until bacon starts getting crispy
5. The color of Tuna starts to fade away, and the bacon continues to sizzle

6. Flip it. Be very cautious because it can fall apart when turning Tuna over
7. Cook to your taste, until done. Medium to medium-rare is suggested
8. Brush with a basting sauce, again
9. Until slicing, sprinkle the Tuna gently with freshly ground black pepper

Nutrition 540 Calories 30g Proteins 8g Fat

Tojo's Bar and Grill Orange Roast Pork Loin Recipe

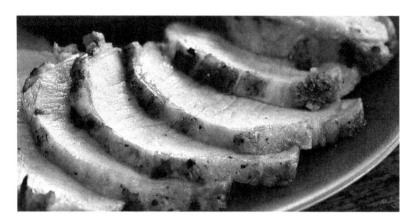

Preparation Time: 24 minutes

Cooking Time: 21 minutes

Servings: 4

Ingredients:

- 12 cups of pork loin
- 2 small oranges, juiced
- 3 tbsp. of fresh rosemary
- 5 cloves sliced of garlic
- 3 tbsp. of olive oil
- Freshly ground black pepper
- Salt
- 2 tbsp. of paprika

Direction

1. Let the oven preheat to 400F

2. Brush the pork with olive oil all over and spritz with sea salt, paprika pepper. Rub the garlic and rosemary on the bacon

3. Mix the liquid ingredients

4. Put the pork loin in a big baking dish, and pour over the pork 1/2 of lime juices

5. Bake for 1 hour in the oven. Place any of the residual juices over the pork loin every 20 minutes, and then turn the pork loin

6. Remove from the oven until pork loin hits 145F at its internal temperature

7. Rest it for a while. Meanwhile, it will keep cooking once it is out from the oven

Nutrition 302 Calories 23g Proteins 16g Fat

SAUCE AND DRESSING RECIPES

Lawry's Seasoned Salt

Preparation Time: 5 minutes

Cooking Time: 0 minute

Serving: 1

Ingredients

- 1 tablespoon salt, or to taste
- 2 teaspoons white sugar
- ¼ teaspoon smoked paprika
- ¼ teaspoon turmeric powder
- ¼ teaspoon onion powder
- ¼ teaspoon garlic powder
- ¼ teaspoon cornstarch

Directions

1. Mix all the spices then store in a glass jar. Keep it dry.

Nutrition 360mg sodium 97 calories18g fat

Chick-Fil-A Sauce

Preparation Time: 5 minutes

Cooking Time: 0 minutes

Serving: 4

Ingredient

- ¼ tsp. onion powder
- ¼ tsp. garlic salt
- ½ tbsp. yellow mustard
- ½ cup mayonnaise
- ¼ tsp. smoked paprika
- ½ tbsp. stevia extract, powdered
- 1 tsp. liquid smoke

Direction

1. With a food processor, incorporate all the ingredients in it, wrap with the lid then process for 30 seconds. Pour the sauce into a bowl then serve.

Nutrition: 183 Calories20g Fats 12g Protein

Burger Sauce

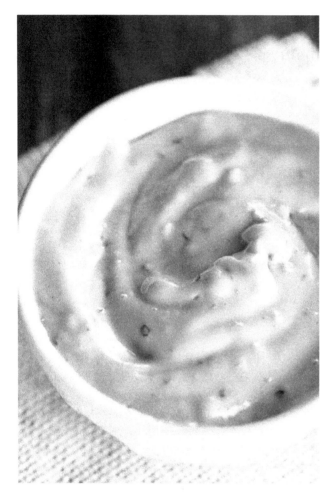

Preparation Time: 5 minutes

Cooking Time: 0 minute

Serving: 12

Ingredient

- 1 tbsp. gherkin
- ½ tsp. chopped dill

- ¾ tsp. onion powder
- ¾ tsp. garlic powder
- 1/8 tsp. ground white pepper
- ½ cup mayonnaise
- 1 tsp. mustard powder
- ½ tsp. erythritol sweetener
- ¼ tsp. sweet paprika
- 1 tsp. white vinegar

Direction

1. Using medium bowl, situate all the ingredients for the sauce in it then stir until well mixed.
2. Situate sauce for a minimum of overnight in the refrigerator to develop flavors and then serve with burgers.

Nutrition: 15 Calories7g Fats2g Protein

Pollo Tropical's Curry Mustard Sauce

Preparation Time: 5 minutes

Cooking Time: 0 minute

Serving: 12

Ingredient:

- 2 tsp. curry powder
- 4 tsp. mustard paste
- 8 tbsp. mayonnaise

Direction:

1. Using a food processor, incorporate all the ingredients in it, then pulse for 30 seconds.
2. Situate into a bowl then serve.

Nutrition: 66 Calories7 g Fats1 g Protein

El Fenix Chili Gravy

Preparation Time: 5 minutes

Cooking Time: 40 minutes

Serving: 28

Ingredient:

- 2 tbsp. coconut flour
- ½ tsp. salt
- ½ tsp. black pepper
- 1/2 tsp. dried Mexican oregano leaves
- ¼ cup lard
- 1 ½ tsp. garlic powder
- 2 tsp. ground cumin
- 2 cups beef broth
- ½ tsp. ground coriander
- 2 tbsp. oat fiber
- 2 tbsp. red chili powder
- 1/8 tsp. dried thyme leaves

Direction

1. Using medium skillet pan, situate it over medium heat, add lard and once melts, stir in flour, and then cook for 4 minutes, regularly lifting the pan from heat to cool slightly and then put it back onto the fire.

2. Mix in oat fiber, garlic, thyme, oregano, cumin, and coriander cook for 2 minutes until it gets thick, stirring constantly.
3. Pour in the broth until smooth, switch heat to the low level, and simmer the gravy fo3 30 minutes until sauce thickens. Remove pan from heat and serve.

Nutrition: 22 Calories2g Fats0.9g Protein

Sweet and Smoky Chipotle Vinaigrette

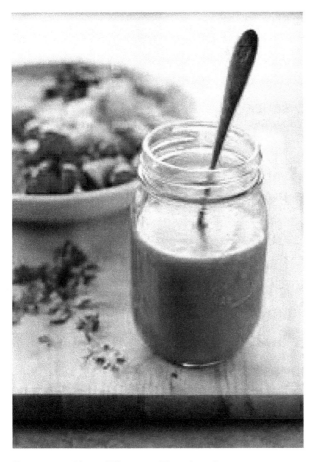

Preparation Time: 5 minutes

Cooking Time: 0 minute

Serving: 32

Ingredient

- 1 tsp. garlic powder
- 1 tsp. cumin

- 1 tbsp. salt
- 1 ½ tbsp. ground black pepper
- 1 tsp. oregano leaves
- 1/3 cup liquid stevia
- ½ cup red wine vinegar
- 1 ½ cups avocado oil
- 1 tbsp. adobo sauce
- 1 tbsp. water

Direction

1. Using food processor, incorporate all the ingredients in it except for oil, close then pulse for 30 seconds.
2. Whisk in oil until mixed and then pour the salad dressing into a medium bowl.
3. Serve straight away.

Nutrition: 103 Calories11.5g Fats0.05g Protein

Bang-Bang Sauce

Preparation Time: 5 minutes

Cooking Time: 0 minute

Serving: 6

Ingredient:

- ¼ cup mayonnaise
- 1 ½ tbsp. garlic chili sauce
- 1 tbsp. rice vinegar
- 2 tbsp. monk fruit Sweetener
- 1/8 tsp. salt

Direction:

1. Using food processor, mix all the ingredients in it, close then pulse for 30 seconds then serve.

Nutrition: 90 Calories 10g Fats 1g Net Carbohydrates

Sweet Chili Sauce

Preparation Time: 5 minutes

Cooking Time: 15 minutes

Serving: 6

Ingredient

- 1 tbsp. garlic chili sauce
- ½ cup of water
- 2 cups of beef bone broth collagen
- 1 tbsp. avocado oil
- ¼ cup unseasoned rice vinegar
- 1 ½ tsp. minced garlic
- ¼ tsp. ground ginger
- ¼ cup erythritol sweetener

Direction

1. Incorporate all the ingredients in it except for oil then whisk well.
2. Using medium saucepan, situate it over medium heat, add sauce mixture then simmer it for 15 minutes.
3. Once done, pull away the pan from heat, stir in oil, let the sauce cool completely and then serve.

Nutrition: 25 Calories 2.2 g Fats 1.2 g Carbohydrates

Big Mac Sauce

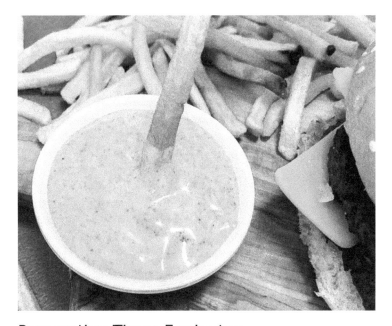

Preparation Time: 5 minutes

Cooking Time: 0 minute

Serving: 6

Ingredient:

- 1 tbsp. diced white onion
- 2 tbsp. diced pickles
- 1 tsp. erythritol sweetener
- 1 tbsp. ketchup, low-carb
- 1 tsp. dill pickle juice
- ½ cup mayonnaise

Direction:

1. Incorporate all of its ingredients in it then stir well.
2. Serve straight away.

Nutrition: 138 Calories 16g Fats 1g Carbohydrates

DESSERT RECIPES

Banana Cream Cheesecake

Preparation Time: 20 minutes

Cooking Time: 1 hour 30 minutes

Servings: 4

Ingredients

- 20 vanilla sandwich cookies
- ¼ cup margarine, melted
- 3 (8-ounce) packages cream cheese, softened
- 2/3 cup granulated sugar
- 2 tablespoons cornstarch
- 3 eggs
- ¾ cup mashed bananas
- ½ cup whipping cream
- 2 teaspoons vanilla extract

Directions

1. Preheat the oven to 350°F. Crumble cookies in blender. When they have turned to crumbs, add the melted butter. Situate mixture in a springform pan and press to entirely cover the

bottom and up the sides of the pan. Refrigerate this.

2. Scourge cream cheese until creamy, and add the sugar and corn starch. When the cheese mixture is well blended, add in the eggs one at a time. When the eggs are incorporated, add the bananas, whipping cream, and vanilla, beating until well combined.

3. Transfer filling into the springform pan and bake at 350°F for 15 minutes. Reduce the heat to 200°F and bake until the center of the cheesecake is set, about 1 hour and 15 minutes.

4. When the center is set, remove the cake from the oven. Pop the spring on the pan, but don't remove the sides until the cheesecake has cooled completely. When it is cool, transfer it to the refrigerator. Refrigerate for at least 4 hours before serving. Serve with whipped cream and freshly sliced bananas.

Nutrition: 46g Carbohydrates 11g fats 5g protein

Blackout Cake

Preparation Time: 30 minutes

Cooking Time: 35–45 minutes

Servings: 8 - 10

Ingredients

For the Cake:

- 1 cup butter, softened
- 4 cups sugar
- 4 large eggs
- 4 teaspoons vanilla extract, divided
- 6 ounces unsweetened chocolate, melted
- 4 cups flour
- 4 teaspoons baking soda
- ½ teaspoon salt
- 1 cup buttermilk
- 1 ¾ cups boiling water

For the Chocolate Ganache:

- 12 ounces semisweet chocolate, chips or chopped
- 3 cups heavy cream
- 4 tablespoons butter, chopped
- 2 teaspoons vanilla
- 1 ½ cups roasted almonds, crushed (for garnish)

Directions

1. Preheat the oven to 350°F. Prep two large rimmed baking sheets with parchment paper

2. In a large bowl or bowl for a stand mixer, beat together the butter and sugar until well combined. When the sugar mixture is fluffy, add the eggs and 2 teaspoons of vanilla. When that is combined, add the 4 ounces of melted chocolate and mix well.

3. In a separate bowl, stir together the flour, baking soda, and salt. Gradually add half the flour mixture to the chocolate mixture. When it is combined, add half of the buttermilk and mix until combined. Repeat with remaining flour mixture and buttermilk. When it is completely combined, add the boiling water and mix thoroughly.

4. Portion batter evenly between the two large baking sheets that you prepared earlier (or 3 8-inch cake pans).

5. Situate to the oven and bake for 20–30 minutes for the baking sheets or 25-35 minutes for the cake pans, or until a toothpick inserted in the center comes out clean.

6. Remove from the oven and let cakes cool for about 10 minutes. With the pastry ring, make 3 cakes from each of the baking sheet. When they

are completely cool down. If using cake pans, turn them out onto a cooling rack and let them cool completely and then cut horizontally into two to make 6 cake layers

7. Make the ganache by mixing the chocolate chips and cream in a heat-safe glass bowl. Situate bowl over a pot of boiling water. Reduce heat to medium-low and let simmer gently. Stir continuously using wooden spoon until the chocolate is all melted. Add-in the butter and vanilla and stir until well combined. Let cool for a few minutes, cover with plastic wrap, and refrigerate until the ganache holds its shape and is spreadable, about 10 minutes.

8. To assemble the cake, place the first cake layer on a serving plate and spread a some of the ganache on the top. Situate second cake layer on top and spread some of the ganache on top. Repeat until all 6 layers are done. With the remaining ganache to frost the top and sides of the cake, then cover the sides with crushed almonds (if desired) by pressing them gently into the chocolate ganache. Refrigerate before serving.

Nutrition: 41g Carbohydrates 10g fats 4g protein

Molten Lava Cake

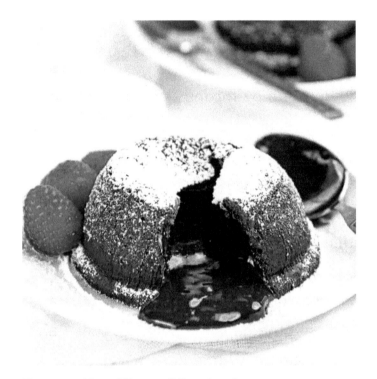

Preparation Time: 20 minutes

Cooking Time: 10 minutes

Servings: 5-6

Ingredients:

For the Cakes:

- Six tablespoons unsalted butter (2 tablespoons melted, four tablespoons at room temperature)
- 1/2 cup natural cocoa powder (not Dutch process), plus more for dusting
- 1 1/3 cups all-purpose flour
- One teaspoon baking soda

- 1/2 teaspoon baking powder
- 1/2 teaspoon salt
- Three tablespoons milk
- 1/4 cup vegetable oil
- 1 1/3 cups sugar
- 1 1/2 teaspoons vanilla extract
- Two large eggs, at room temperature

For the Fillings and Toppings:

- 8 ounces bittersweet chocolate, finely chopped
- 1/2 cup heavy cream
- Four tablespoons unsalted butter
- One tablespoon light corn syrup
- Caramel sauce, for drizzling
- 1-pint vanilla ice cream

Directions:

1. Oven preheats to 350 degrees F. Make the cakes: Brush four one 1/4-cup brioche molds (jumbo muffin cups or 10-ounce ramekins) with the butter melted in 2 tablespoons. Clean the cocoa powdered molds and tap the excess.

2. In a small bowl, whisk in the flour, baking soda, baking powder, and salt. Bring 3/4 cup water& the milk and over medium heat to a boil in a saucepan; set aside.

3. Use a stand mixer, combine vegetable oil, four tablespoons of room-temperature butter and sugar and beat with the paddle attachment until it's fluffy at medium-high speed, around 4 minutes, scrape the bowl down and beat as desired. Add 1/2 cup cocoa powder and vanilla; beat over medium velocity for 1 minute. Scrape the pot beneath. Add one egg and beat at medium-low speed for 1 minute, then add the remaining egg and beat for another minute.

4. Gradually beat in the flour mixture with the mixer on a low level, then the hot milk mixture. Finish combining the batter with a spatula of rubber before mixed. Divide the dough equally between the molds, each filling slightly more than three-quarters of the way.

5. Move the molds to a baking sheet and bake for 25 to 30 minutes, until the tops of the cakes feel domed, and the centers are just barely set. Move the baking sheet to a rack; allow the cakes to cool for about 30 minutes before they pull away from the molds.

6. How to set up the Cake: Make the Filling: Microwave the sugar, butter, chocolate, and corn syrup in a microwave-safe bowl at intervals of 30

seconds, stirring each time, until the chocolate starts to melt, 1 minute, 30 seconds. Let sit for three minutes and then whisk until smooth. Reheat, if possible, before use.

7. Using a paring knife tip to remove the cakes gently from the molds, then invert the cakes onto a cutting board.

8. Hollow out a spoon to the cake; save the scraps. Wrap the plastic wrap and microwave cakes until steaming, for 1 minute.

9. Drizzle the caramel plates, unwrap the cakes then put them on top. Pour three tablespoons into each cake filling.

10. Plug in a cake scrap to the door. Save any leftover scraps or discard them.

11. Top each cake, use an ice cream scoop. Spoon more chocolate sauce on top, spread thinly so that it is coated in a jar.

Nutrition: 546 Calories 5g Protein 31g Fat

White Chocolate Raspberry Nothing Bundt Cakes

Preparation Time: 20 minutes

Cooking Time: 10 minutes

Servings: 5-6

Ingredients:

- Chopped into small cubes, 200g butter, plus extra for greasing
- 100g white chocolate, broken into pieces
- Four large eggs
- 200g caster sugar
- 200g self-rising flour
- 175g raspberries, fresh or frozen
- For the ganache
- 200g white chocolate, chopped
- 250ml double cream
- A little icing sugar, for dusting

Directions:

1. Heat oven to fan/gas 4, 180C/160C. Grease and line the 2 x 20 cm round base with loose-bottomed cake tins. In a heat-proof mixing bowl, place the butter and chocolate, set over a pan of

barely simmering water, and allow to melt gradually, stirring occasionally.

2. Once butter and chocolate have melted, remove from heat and cool for 1-2 minutes, then beat with an electric whisk in the eggs and sugar. Fold and raspberries in the starch.

3. Pour the mixture gently into the tins and bake for 20-25 minutes. Pullout the cakes from the oven & allow for 10 minutes of cooling in the tins before placing on a wire rack.

4. To make the ganache, place the chocolate over a pan of barely simmering water in a heatproof bowl with 100ml of the cream on top. Remove until the chocolate has melted into the sugar, and leave a smooth, shiny ganache on you. You need to leave the ganache at room temperature to cool, then beat in the rest of the cream.

5. Sandwich them together with the chocolate ganache after the cakes have cooled. Just before serving, sprinkle them with icing sugar.

Nutrition: 489 Calories 3.9g Protein 28g Fat

Caramel Rockslide Brownies

Preparation Time: 25 minutes

Cooking Time: 25 minutes

Servings: 5-6

Ingredients:

- 1 cup butter (2 sticks)
- 2 cups of sugar
- Four eggs
- Two teaspoons vanilla extract
- 2/3 cup unsweetened natural cocoa powder
- 1 cup all-purpose flour
- 1/2 teaspoon salt
- One teaspoon baking powder
- 1/2 cup semisweet chocolate chips
- 1 cup (plus more for drizzling over the top) caramel topping
- 3/4 cup chopped pecans (plus more for sprinkling on top)

Directions:

1. Preheat to 350 degrees on the oven. On a medium saucepan melt butter over medium heat.
2. Clear from heat the pan and whisk in sugar. Whisk in the vanilla extract & the eggs. Mix the cocoa, baking powder, flour, salt, and in a

separate dish. Drop the dry ingredients into the saucepan and combine them until they have just been added. Add chocolate chips.

3. Pour the batter into two nine by 9-inch baking pans that are evenly split, sprayed with nonstick spray and lined with parchment paper.

4. Bake for 25-28 minutes and leave to cool.

5. Use the parchment paper edges to lift the whole brownie out of one of the pans, and chop into 1/2-inch cubes.

6. Pour 1 cup of caramel over the brownies still in the saucepan, then add the chopped pecans and brownie cubes.

7. Press down to make the caramel stick to the brownie cubes. If desired, drizzle with extra caramel and sprinkle with a few more chopped pecans.

8. If needed, serve with ice cream and excess sugar, and chopped pecans.

Nutrition: 509 Calories 5g Protein 32g Fat

Cornbread Muffins

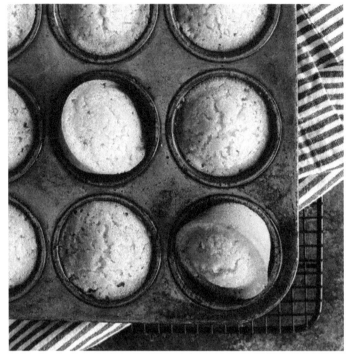

Preparation

Time: 10 minutes

Cooking Time: 25 minutes

Servings: 6-7

Ingredients:

- ½ cup butter softened
- 2/3 Cup white sugar
- ¼ cup honey
- Two eggs
- ½ teaspoon salt
- 1 ½ cups all-purpose flour

- ¾ cup cornmeal
- ½ teaspoon baking powder
- ½ cup milk
- ¾ cup frozen corn kernels, thawed

Directions:

1. Preheat oven to 400 grades F (200 grades C). Grease or 12 cups of muffins on deck.

2. Cream the butter, sugar, honey, eggs, and salt together in a big pot. Add in rice, cornmeal, and baking powder, blend well. Stir in corn and milk. Pour the yield into prepared muffin cups or spoon them.

3. Bake for 20 to 25 minutes in a preheated oven until a toothpick inserted in the center of a muffin comes out clean.

Nutrition: 141 Calories 6g Protein 18g Fat

Chocolate Mousse Cake

Preparation Time: 10 minutes

Cooking Time: 25 minutes

Servings: 6-7

Ingredients:

- 1 (18.25 ounce) chocolate cake mix pack
- 1 (14 ounces) can sweeten condensed milk
- 2 (1 ounce) squares unsweetened chocolate, melted
- ½ cup of cold water
- 1 (3.9 ounces) package instant chocolate pudding mix
- 1 cup heavy cream, whipped

Directions:

1. Preheat oven up to 175 degrees C (350 degrees F). Prepare and bake cake mix on two 9-inch layers according to package directions. Cool off and pan clean.
2. Mix the sweetened condensed milk and melted chocolate together in a big tub. Stir in water slowly, then pudding instantly until smooth. Chill in for 30 minutes, at least.
3. Remove from the fridge the chocolate mixture, and whisk to loosen. Fold in the whipped cream

and head back to the refrigerator for at least another hour.

4. Place one of the cake layer onto a serving platter. Top the mousse with 1 1/2 cups, then cover with the remaining cake layer. Frost with remaining mousse, and cool until served. Garnish with chocolate shavings or fresh fruit.

Nutrition: 324 Calories 8g Protein 50g Fat

Blackberry and Apples Cobbler

Preparation Time: 10 minutes

Cooking Time: 30 minutes

Servings: 6

Ingredients:

- ¾ cup stevia
- 6 cups blackberries
- ¼ cup apples, cored and cubed
- ¼ teaspoon baking powder
- 1 tablespoon lime juice
- ½ cup almond flour
- ½ cup of water
- 3 and ½ tablespoon avocado oil
- Cooking spray

Directions:

1. In a bowl, mix the berries with half of the stevia and lemon juice, sprinkle some flour all over, whisk and pour into a baking dish greased with cooking spray.
2. In another bowl, mix flour with the rest of the sugar, baking powder, the water and the oil, and stir the whole thing with your hands.
3. Spread over the berries, introduce in the oven at 375° F and bake for 30 minutes. Serve warm.

Nutrition: 221 Calories 6.3g Fat 9g Protein

Black Tea Cake

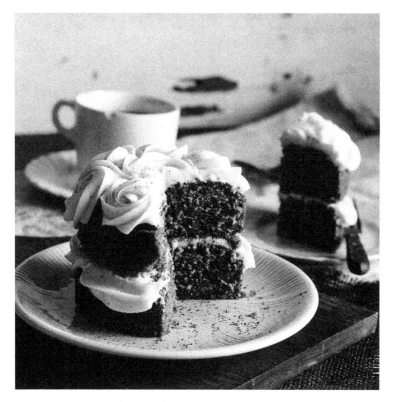

Preparation Time: 10 minutes

Cooking Time: 35 minutes

Servings: 8

Ingredients:

- 6 tablespoons black tea powder
- 2 cups almond milk, warmed up
- 1 cup avocado oil
- 2 cups stevia
- 4 eggs
- 2 teaspoons vanilla extract

- 3 and ½ cups almond flour
- 1 teaspoon baking soda
- 3 teaspoons baking powder

Directions:

1. Blend almond milk with the oil, stevia and the rest of the ingredients and whisk well.
2. Pour this into a cake pan lined with parchment paper, introduce in the oven at 350° F and bake for 35 minutes. Leave the cake to cool down, slice and serve.

Nutrition: 200 Calories 6.4g Fat 5.4g Protein

Quinoa Muffins

Preparation Time: 10 minutes

Cooking Time: 30 minutes

Servings: 12

Ingredients:

- 1 cup quinoa, cooked
- 6 eggs, whisked
- Salt and black pepper to the taste
- 1 cup Swiss cheese, grated
- 1 small yellow onion, chopped
- 1 cup white mushrooms, sliced
- ½ cup sun-dried tomatoes, chopped

Directions:

1. In a bowl, combine the eggs with salt, pepper and the rest of the ingredients and whisk well.
2. Divide this into a silicone muffin pan, bake at 350 degrees F for 30 minutes and serve for breakfast.

Nutrition: 123 Calories 5.6g Fat 7.5g Protein

Figs Pie

Preparation Time: 10 minutes

Cooking Time: 1 hour

Servings: 8

Ingredients:

- ½ cup stevia
- 6 figs, cut into quarters
- ½ teaspoon vanilla extract
- 1 cup almond flour
- 4 eggs, whisked

Directions:

1. Spread the figs on the bottom of a spring form pan lined with parchment paper.
2. In a bowl, combine the other ingredients, whisk and pour over the figs,
3. Bake at 375° F for 1 hour, flip the pie upside down when it's done and serve.

Nutrition: 200 Calories 4.4g Fat 8g Protein

BEVERAGE RECIPES

Sangarita

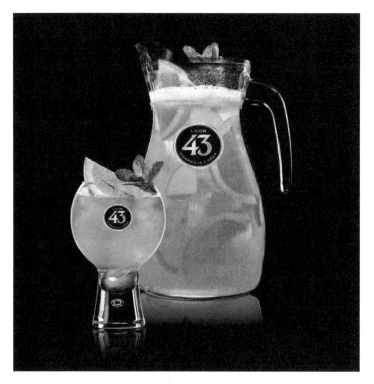

Preparation Time: 10 minutes

Cooking Time: 10 minutes

Servings: 10

Ingredients

- 10 ounces grenadine
- 2 bottles red table wine
- 16 ounces cranberry juice cocktail

- 10 ounces simple syrup (5 ounces sugar dissolved in 5 ounces water)
- 12 ounces sweet vermouth
- Strawberries & oranges, sliced
- crushed ice

Directions

1. Mix everything together (except ice) in a large pitcher. Pour the sangria in 10 glasses & then add some crushed ice into each glass. Fill each glass with sliced strawberries and oranges.

Nutrition: 51 Calories 10g Protein 4g Fat

Limoncello Lemonade

Preparation Time: 10 minutes

Cooking Time: 10 minutes

Servings: 1

Ingredients

- 4 teaspoons lemon juice
- ¼ cup granulated sugar
- 1-ounce citrus-infused vodka, Smirnoff
- 4 ounces lemonade concentrate
- 1-ounce Limoncello liqueur, lemon-flavored liqueur
- ¼ cup hot water
- 1 -2 cup ice

Directions

1. Combine sugar with lemon juice & hot water and prepare the lemon syrup; set aside at room temperature to cool.
2. When cool, prepare the drink by combining ¼ ounce of the lemon syrup with lemonade, Limoncello, citrus vodka and ice in a blender. Blend until the ice is crushed, on high speed.
3. Begin with one cup of ice & add more of ice to make the drink slushy, if required. Pour the drink

in a 16-ounce glass and garnish the glass with a thin slice of lemon. Serve & enjoy.

Nutrition: 41 Calories 12g Protein 5g Fat

Lemonade

Preparation Time: 1 minute

Cooking Time: 0 minutes

Servings 1

Ingredients

- 1-quart water
- 1 cup sugar
- 1 cup fresh lemon juice
- Sparkling water (not tonic water)

Directions

1. Mix the water, sugar, and lemon juice together.

2. Fill a glass 2/3 to ¾ full of the lemon mixture (depending on your preference) and top it off with sparkling water.

3. You can change the flavor of the lemonade by adding puréed fruit (raspberries, strawberries, etc.). You may want to add a bit more sugar if you are adding fresh fruit.

Nutrition: 150 Calories 0.1g Fat 0.2g Protein

Margarita

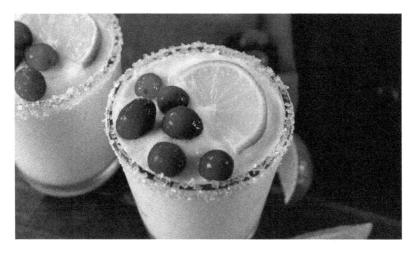

Preparation Time: 1 minute

Cooking Time: 0 minutes

Servings 1

Ingredients

- 1 ½ ounces Cuervo or 1800 gold tequila
- ¾ ounce Cointreau
- ¾ ounce Grand Marnier
- ½ ounce lime juice
- 2 ounces sour mix
- Ice, for serving

Directions

1. Refrigerate (or even freeze) the glass you intend to use.

2. While chilling, mix together all the ingredients in a shaker and shake well.

3. If you like salt on the rim of your margarita, pour some sea salt on a small dish, wet the rim of your chilled glass, and dip into the salt.

4. Add some ice, and pour the margarita mixture in.

Nutrition: 153 Calories 2g Fat 0.2g Protein

Iced Green Tea Latte

Preparation Time: 2 minutes

Cooking Time: 0 minutes

Servings: 1

Ingredients

- 3 cups milk
- 2 teaspoons matcha powder
- 2 tablespoons water
- 2-3 teaspoons honey
- 1 teaspoon vanilla extract
- Ice

Directions

1. Mix matcha powder and water. Stir until there are no clumps.
2. Incorporate milk, matcha mixture, vanilla extract, and honey. Stir or shake in a covered container until well combined.
3. Divide into two cups and serve over ice.

Nutrition: 226 Calories 7g Fat 13g Protein

Orange Julius

Preparation time: 10 minutes

Cooking Time: 0 minutes

Servings: 2

Ingredients

- 1½ cups milk, skim milk
- 1 teaspoon vanilla extract
- 1 cup frozen orange juice concentrate
- 1/3 cup superfine sugar
- 1 cup ice cubes

Directions

1. Take a blender and pulse together vanilla extract and milk.
2. Add sugar, ice, and orange juice concentrate.
3. Blend well.
4. Once thickened, pour the mixture into serving glasses and enjoy.

Nutrition: 161 Calories 1.8g fat 3.3g Protein

Snapple Lemon Iced Tea

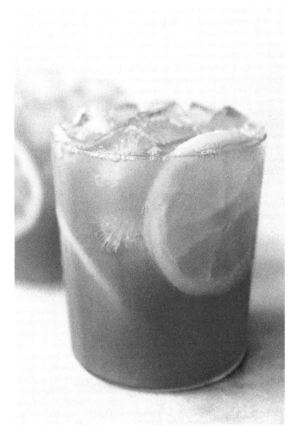

Preparation time: 5 minutes

Cooking Time: 0 minutes

Servings: 5

Ingredients

- 10 cups water
- 4 teabags Lipton black tea
- ½ cup white sugar
- 1 cup lemon juice

Directions

1. Get saucepan and bring the water to a boil.

2. Add teabags and let sit for 1 hour.

3. Add sugar and stir well.

4. Pour this mixture into the pitcher.

5. Add lemon juice and chill in the refrigerator for 6 hours.

6. Once chilled, serve.

Nutrition: 87 Calories 0.4g fat 0.2g Protein

Hawaiian Punch Red

Preparation time: 10 minutes

Cooking Time: 0 minutes

Servings: 5

Ingredients

- 2 cups filtered water
- 2 cups fresh pineapple juice
- ½ cup guava/passion fruit blend
- ½ cup fresh orange juice
- ½ cup fresh apple juice
- ½ cup papaya nectar
- ½ cup apricot nectar
- ¼ cup white superfine sugar
- ½ teaspoon red food coloring
- Ice cubes, orange slices, and cherries for serving

Directions

1. Combine all the ingredients in a pitcher.
2. Stir and serve once dissolved in a glass full of ice cubes. Decorate with orange slices and cherries if desired.

Nutrition: 150 Calories 0.5g fat 1.2g Protein

All-Natural Lemonade

Preparation time: 10 minutes

Cooking Time: 0 minutes

Servings: 2

Ingredients

- ½ cup fresh lemon juice
- 1/3 cup granulated sugar
- 3 cups water

Directions

1. Combine all the ingredients in a pitcher.
2. Stir to combine well.
3. Chill for 2 hours and serve.

Nutrition: 140 Calories 0.5g fat 0.5g Protein

Ginseng and Honey Green Tea

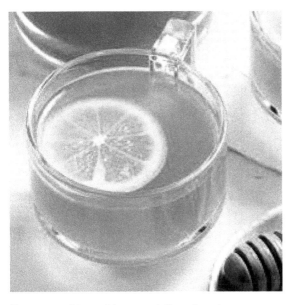

Preparation time: 10 minutes

Cooking Time: 0 minutes

Servings: 1

Ingredients

- 10 cups water
- 3 green tea teabags
- ½ cup superfine sugar
- 2 tablespoons honey
- 2 tablespoons lemon juice
- ½ teaspoon American ginseng extract
- Ice cubes and lemon slices for serving

Directions

1. Take a large saucepan and boil water in it.
2. Turn off the heat and add tea bags and sugar to the water. Mix well until sugar has dissolved. Add remaining ingredients. Stir to combine.
3. Cover and steep the tea bags for one hour at room temperature. Discard teabags and place in the refrigerator until ready to serve, at least 1 hour.
4. Serve chilled over ice cubes with lemon slices if desired.

Nutrition 116 Calories 0.2g fat 0.1g Protein

CONCLUSION

Creativity often happens when you cook at home, and you can attach a range of plant foods to a variety of colors. The copycat recipes are perfect for the dishes you want to recreate.

But, watch out. Everyone has their favorite dishes, and others love to have a bite of their world-famous recipes. Will you be the first to make a copycat recipe that tastes the same as the original recipe? Or will you mix in the wrong ingredients, and damage the recipe so that you end up with a concoction that tastes weird?

You need to have all your ingredients collection, mix them up and see how you can make the taste just like the original recipe.

Serving control from home can be regulated. Once the food is cooked for us, we tend to eat all or most of it. Try to use little dishes at home, but ensure that all good things like vegetables, fruits, whole grains, and legumes are filled. You are certainly going to be satisfied and happy.

The major advantage of trying copycat restaurant recipes is that you can save more money and use your creativity to improve the dish. You can also adjust the ingredients and add those favorite herbs to your desired taste. Now you have saved your money and restaurant-quality dishes for your family as well.

You may not include some ingredients of your favorite dish when you try the copycat recipes, and it is okay. Following the recipe while recreating your favorite dish is what we are here for.

It is not hard to acquire those top-secret restaurant-quality recipes. Others may advise that you need to have culinary credentials to cook those secret recipes. Yet, we can gather those ingredients ourselves and cook an elaborate meal that tastes like the real deal.

But do top secret restaurant recipes taste the way the chef served them? Perhaps. You can easily recreate your favorite recipes with patience and a little practice. You may start to think that some recipes need additional seasonings to improve your dish than the original. Nevertheless, if you wanted to prepare this dish on your own, there is still a chance.

Just a few simple tips and tricks, you can also make quality cuisine in your kitchen. These tricks may not seem so strong on their own but can transform how you prepare and produce food when they are all used together. These tips help you cook at home like a pro from expired spices and how you use salt to arrange it before you start cooking.

When preparing desserts at home, you can tweak the recipes as you wish. As you sample the recipes, you will know the usual ingredients and techniques in making popular sweet treats. It could inspire you to create your very own recipes. You can use alternative ingredients according to your taste, budget or health. You can come up, possibly, not with a dish that is perfectly alike as the restaurant's recipe, but with one that is exactly the way you want it to be. Most of all, the recipes here are meant for you to experience the contentment of seeing those smiles on the people whom you share with your dishes or creations. Keep cooking and have fun with the recipes, and soon, you will be reaping your sweet rewards!

If prepared food reaches outside the home, you typically have limited knowledge about salt, sugar, and processed oils. For a fact, we also apply more to our meal when it is served to the table. You will say how much salt, sugar, and oil are being used to prepare meals at home.

Copycat recipes practically give you the ability to make great restaurant food tasting in your own home and get it the right first time and easily.

CPSIA information can be obtained
at www.ICGtesting.com
Printed in the USA
BVHW052027120421
604747BV00005B/339